Swimming for the Mature Person

Swimming for the Mature Person

Donald Lewis MacKeen

Published by MacKeen Consultants Inc

ISBN: 978-1-257-93529

Contents

Introduction and forward

This self-teaching booklet was written for mature persons who either do not swim or do not swim well, and rarely exercise. Recall the countless times you have thought about doing something to correct this situation; until today you've done nothing. There was always been a good reason to put it off. We all recognize the excuses: It would be embarrassing to take swimming instruction where everyone else, including the instructor, is young and trim; individual instruction would be too expensive; water in the eyes causes panic because of a near drowning years ago (my main excuse); there is a medical or physical condition that might cause difficulty; or, last but not least, the times or places where the lessons are held are never convenient.

Prior to my active involvement in swimming, I was seeking an appropriate exercise for weight loss. I'd quit jogging because of knee and hip discomfort, and my golf game had gotten worse than you could imagine. I had spoken many times about taking swimming lessons as I had access to a pool, but had done nothing. My wife recognized my predicament and borrowed a book on swimming from the local library. It provided me with a single clue that enabled me to begin swimming; I was then only 60. After ten years of regular swimming I was so fit that I sailed through and recuperated quickly from a series of major surgeries (none caused by swimming).

This booklet offers self-instruction you can tailor to your time and situation; I have added related comments and suggestions which I feel are appropriate, and potentially helpful. The method is simple and effective. It worked for me, it can work for you. The lessons cover only one style of swimming, after you have learned these methods, modify them if you wish to better suit your needs and goals.

Initially the development of this series of lesson was an unplanned series of events which began when I learned how to breathe while swimming. This vital shred of instruction gleaned from the library book was the only outside instruction I have knowingly utilized. It opened my eyes (goggled, of course) and resulted in my being more at home in the water. From then on my approach to learning and improving my swimming was quite simple: I wanted to swim smoothly and as rapidly as possible with minimal exertion. These goals were enabled and limited by movement of my arms and legs and the positioning of my body. I considered, tested, honed and then applied various ways to improve my new-found sport; this was all done within the limits of my age-related capabilities.

Exercise improves our circulations, a status that is lessened during hours of inactivity while reading or watching TV.

Your circulation may be worse than you realize until you see the results of the following simple test. Pick up a small flap of skin from the back of your hand using thumb and forefinger; release it. The flap should disappear immediately on release. I'm sure it will not. This experiment will reveal the diminished status of circulation in the many organs of your entire body by testing the largest organ, the skin. After a few weeks of swimming you will note an improved test time indicating a better circulation in your skin and presumably in other tissues and organs. In addition to improved blood flow, exercise also increases the production of synovial fluid (joint lubricants). A recent article reports the benefits of swimming among appropriate exercises for those with osteoarthritis (Landro, Laura. "Doctors' New Advice for Joint Pain: Get Moving."WSJ, 12 April 2011: D1+).

When you are lying in water your position and near weightlessness minimize pressure on your joints, especially on the ever-thinning disks separating your vertebral bones (the compression and resultant thinning of these discs while standing or sitting is a major reason why we become shorter and shorter).

I have found physical and mental benefits from swimming. It trimmed me down, did away with joint aches, lowered my glucose readings and renewed a pleasant relationship with many long- forgotten muscles. It renewed the firmness of my abdominal muscles – much needed after multiple surgeries. Finally, there are psychological benefits: Each session can be an enjoyable period when you are alone with your thoughts, temporarily free of phone calls, faxes or other disruptions. It has even improved my disposition (so my wife says).

Goals and Benefits

The main goal is for you to enjoy swimming gracefully and almost effortlessly. It can leave you refreshed without muscle or joint aches. Gradually you will look and feel better; your skin and muscle tone as well as your weight and vital signs can be improved. It might even improve your disposition too, if needed.

SECTION 1: Preliminary information for all involved

First, see your primary care physician before starting this or any other exercise program. Describe your plan to start a regular routine of swimming. The response given you may include certain limitations on exertion and possibly include some follow-up exercises unique to your condition. Ask for your recommended maximum heart rate (MHR) value; a number you should keep track of during exercise.

Maximum heart rate is calculated differently for swimmers. MHR is calculated differently for swimmers. One way of determining it is provided by Kevin Polansky: www.howtobefit.com/heart-rate-monitoring-part-one.htm. The calculation is simple and assumes that the maximum heart rates are 226 and 220 for men and women respectively. To determine your maximum heart rate by his method subtract your age and the value 10 (value 10 is in the the equation I'm told because the heart does less work while the body is in water). For example the MHR for a 50 year old woman would be 220-50-10 = 160. When starting exercise, he recommends limiting the rate during exertion to 50-60% of the calculated value; in this example the initial maximum initial heart rate should be 96 beats per minute (60% of 160).

It is imperative, especially during the initial lessons to check and recheck the status of your heart. This should be done at the end of laps during each session to assure you do not exceed your maximum heart rate (MHR). You can do this with either with a wrist heart rate monitor (cost is $40+/- on the internet) or by counting it. This latter determination can be made by timing it with your water-proof wristwatch or the clock available at many pools. Check it from time to time at the end of a lap by placing your finger tips gently over the artery located on the inner side of your arm's radius bone (the one on the thumb side) where it joins the hand) and count the beats per minute. A simpler, approximate determination can be made by counting the beats during five second interval. For example, five beats in five seconds is a heart rate of 60, 10 beats is a rate of 120, etc. If you have concerns about rhythm irregularities, time it for longer periods then discuss your findings with your doctor.

You will be able to determine if your current physical status is improving or not by comparing your original resting pulse rate with that after a few weeks of exercise. If your morning rate is slower it implies you are improving physically. However, if your resting rate has increased it appears you are either over-exercising or possibly are coming down with a cold or other problem; regardless of the cause you should slow down temporarily. As you improve based on your new resting heart rate and swimming speed, you may decide to gradually increase your MHR up to the recommended value of 80-90%.

Second, you will need reasonable access to a pool, lake or ocean. If convenient you might join a nearby Y that has a pool; check on the internet for nearby sites. If I were searching and found several available pools, I would select the one that uses ozone or UV for water disinfection and is heated during cold periods. When no pools are available, consider having a pool built when it meets your available space and budget. When space is limited, investigate having either a one- or two-lane lap pool built or purchase a small indoor in which you swim against an oncoming flow of water.

Third, be sure that you have the correct equipment. Purchase a snorkel mask with breathing tube, swim goggles and, of course, a swimsuit. Select quality equipment; apparent bargains often have drawbacks in terms of comfort and durability. And do not forget to purchase sun block to protect your skin from repeated exposure to sunlight. Apply it prior to each exposure. Be aware you can burn even on overcast days. More on this is in

Section 6.

Fourth, do warm-up exercises. The following exercises can warm your muscles and increase local blood flow. After warming, muscles stretch and contract better and with greater force; blood travels to them faster, and as noted the production of synovial fluid (joint lubricants) is improved.

The exercise is quite simple: Rotate your arms in sequential up and down circular motions similar to those you will make while swimming. The right and left arms copy and follow each other's path in the air.

Start by holding the right arm over your head and the left one down by your hip. Swing the right hand down in front of your face, continue in a curve in front of your chest, and then down by the right side of your waist past your hip; then you will bend that arm and move it back to the starting position above your head. You will have competed a cycle for the right arm. Starting at the same time, bend your left arm up and then extend it as far as possible over your head. Swing your hand in front of your face; continue in a curve in front of your chest and down by the left side of your waist past your hip.

Repeat the cycles. Follow the forward move of each arm with its shoulder, by pivoting your upper body.

This will stretch and warm the back and arm muscles. Do ten or twenty of these depending on your ability. If you are self-conscious about being on display while doing warm-ups, perform them at home before heading to swim, but do them.

Also do deep knee bends or chair stands, especially before swimming in cold water. If you are young, i.e., 50ish or less, try doing deep knee bends. If you are older, you might try chair stands, which is just as it sounds: Stand up from a chair five times as fast as you can.

If any warm-up or swimming movement suggested in the course of this booklet causes discomfort or pain, stop doing it. Use your imagination, when you find a comfortable replacement move, go for it. When you're in your twenties the saying, "No pain, no gain!" may be wise counsel, but if one is considerably older, pain or discomfort is probably your body advising you to slow down or stop. Heed that message, if you don't, you may do temporary or even permanent physical damage to yourself. Self-inflicted damage should not be a goal of this or any other rational sport.

SECTION 2 Primary instruction for non-swimmers & those fearful of water

Introduction

This introductory section is intended for either those who have never swum and/or those who have a fear of breathing while their faces are even partially submerged under water. At this moment you may find it difficult to believe, but swimming is natural. Consider how automatically infants swim before they are old enough to realize that water is different than air.

For your first try wear a snorkel mask fitted with a breathing tube. This is a useful device for certain underwater activities which are not limited to today's lesson. For example you may use it again in subsequent lessons; and later on at places with coral reefs or other interesting underwater sights.

Whenever using a mask or goggles, wet their insides, especially the lenses, as well as the part of your face where they will make contact; this will enhance the creation of a water-tight seal. I prefer to use regular tap water with its minimal chlorine concentration for this because I have sensitive eyes; but for many chlorinated pool water is suitable. Then pour in very small amount of diluted (1:10 or greater) baby shampoo sufficient to just coat the inner surface of each wetted lens. This can create a thin, fully transparent film which can prevent fogging and enhance lens transparency. You might find it useful to carry a small amount of the diluted shampoo in a small container, e.g., a refilled hotel room shampoo bottle, with your swim gear.

Attach the breathing tube to the snorkel mask by its strap. Put it on and press gently on both sides of the frame to cause a little suction between it and your face, you will detect it by the slight pulling sensation around your eyes. Make sure that the straps are flat against your head; twisted straps can prevent creation of a seal.

Preliminary Lesson

The purpose of the following modified warm-up exercise is to speed your ability to breathe while swimming. To do this you need use only the warm-up exercise plus a few added moves that combine deliberate inhalings and exhalings. It is not complex; after practicing you should be ready to duplicate these dry-land- moves while in the water.

The added movements are side-to-side turns of your neck timed with the upward forward swings of each arm. For example, when your right elbow bends and the arm moves up, you will have turned your face so your mouth faces it on the right; that's when you inhale. Repeat with the left arm, etc. After each inhaling start turning your head toward the other side while exhaling, then inhaling when your mouth faces the other arm.

The steps are described below.

Practice the following in air

The following directions are presented in sets for clarity. The events in each set occur simultaneously. There are no stops between the sets; the events are continuous.

- Stretch your right hand over your head, your left hand below your hip. Point your face forward. Exhale.

- Swing your right hand in front of your face, chest and by your waist. Bend your left elbow and swing your arm up. Turn your face (mouth) to your left. Inhale.

- Continue to move your left arm up over your head as far as possible. Start turning your head to the right while exhaling. Bring your right hand down past your hip.

- Start drawing your left hand down. Bend your right elbow and raise your right arm up. Move your head so your mouth faces right; inhale.

Practice these moves until they become automatic.

Practice the following in the water

With the snorkel mask and breathing tube on, stand in the water and bend until your face is immersed. Bite gently on and breathe through the mouth piece. Once you have convinced yourself that you can breathe through this apparatus, stretch out with your face in the water. Congratulations, you are breathing and floating with your face in water; and doing this without wearing any arm or body floatation gear. The main point of this exercise is mental: You realize that you are floating. Now accept that you can float and breathe without any special equipment other than the mask and breathing tube.

Now replace the snorkel mask and breathing tube with goggles for the following introductory lesson in the water. (The lesson uses the same segmented format for clarity; each set shows simultaneous actions, the sets are continuous.)

- Leak-free goggles in place, take a breath and lie face down in the water.

- Stretch your right hand out in front of your head and your left hand back past your hip. Plunge your right hand in the water; pull it backwards in a gentle curve below your face and chest. Turn your face to the left while exhaling gently through your nostrils.

- Bend your left arm, raise it up out of the water and forward. Turn your mouth into the air toward your left arm. Inhale

- Move your left hand forward over and past your head. Turn your face back into the water to your right; exhale gently through your nostrils. Continue to move your right arm toward your hip.

- Plunge your left hand into the water to start its downward stroke. Bend your right arm and lift it up and forward into the air. Move your mouth into the air on the right. Breathe.

- Continue moving your right arm up past your head in preparation for the next stroke. Turn your face back into the water; continue turning your neck to the left while exhaling. At this time push your left hand past your hip.

- Start the stroke by plunging your right hand into the water. Bring your left hand up and out of the water. Turn your head so your mouth is in the air on the left side. Breathe. Your right hand is by your waist.

Finish your left hand's reach above your head and your right hand's push down past your hip.

COMMENTS

The pushing movements of your arms are continuous. When you complete pushing one arm through the water, you start the other. Notice that your mouth is always positioned in the air to inhale near your arm you raised to start its stroke. These events continue from side to side. After practice, see how simply and efficiently you breathe while swimming. As with all these steps: Practice, practice, practice; it will become second nature.

If you have a problem recall you are going through the same basic warm-up moves modified only by the side to side rotation of your head and mouth (and of course, inhaling and exhaling). If necessary repeat the exercise on dry ground; then try it again in the water. Keep in mind - you will float.

Did part of your head not remain in the water while you swam? This may have resulted from a minor problem. I offer two possible solutions. If you cannot exhale through your nostrils do it through pursed lips; if you cannot turn your neck to breathe on both sides, breathe on only one side. If you found the sensation of your legs dragging in the water annoying, purchase a set of small, buoyant plastic devices, called pull buoys, from a swim shop or on the internet. When held between your calves, they will keep your legs level with your body while you practice.

When these moves have become automatic; add the following minor changes to them. When you plunge your hand into the water to start the stroke, hold your fingers at right angles to the palm of your hand; press your thumb against your forefinger. This gives your hand a cup-shape that enables you to start your stroke more easily. Finally, remember to continue your stroke back as far as comfortably possible to gain all the potential propulsion available.

SECTION 3 First lesson for new and current swimmers: plus comments and correction of old habits

Introductory Comments

For those who can swim and have no problem turning their necks, I have some comments before you proceed. To some of you much of this may be redundant, review it anyway and be sure to read the comments at the end of this section; there may be at least one nugget in it.

Keep part of your head in the water at all times while you are swimming. It is much easier than bobbing your head and neck in and out and should eliminate neck strain. If you developed this bad habit, it may take you some time to rid yourself of it; and there are benefits besides the lessened effort and smoother appearance. For example when you follow the method advocated here you present your head to the on-coming water as a nearly constant rocket-shaped (hydrodynamic) surface which lessens drag. Note how it flows around my head and face in Fig. 1 below. It enhanced my "inhaling space".

Breathing while swimming requires a simple maneuver: rotate your head from side to side in time with your arms' strokes. Raise both your mouth and an arm in the air on the same side at the same time. Your lungs have room, previously you exhaled much of your breath into the water.

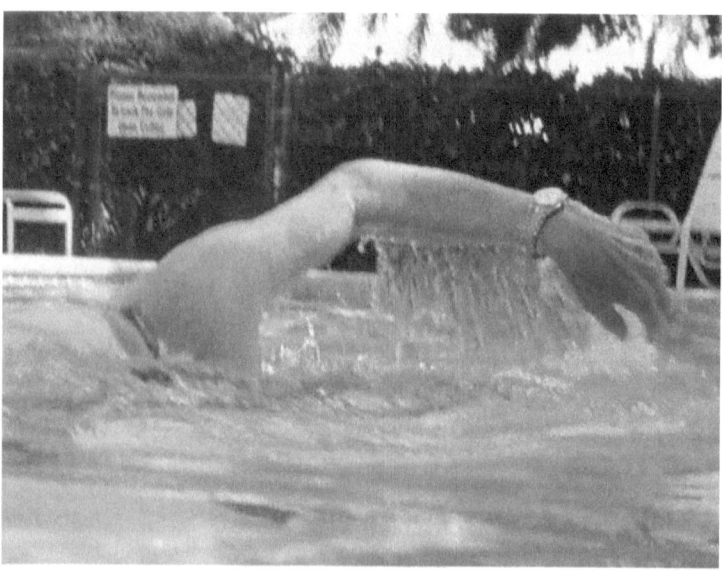

Figure 1: Photograph by Patricia Davies MacKeen

As you continue moving your arm forward past your head, you will turn your face back under water in the opposite direction. While rotating your head toward the other side you will again exhale much of your breath to make room for the next intake. Exhaling is best done through your nostrils, or if that is a problem, through pursed lips.

LESSON

After warm-ups, with leak-tested goggles in place follow these simple steps:

The following directions are presented in sets for clarity. The events in each set occur simultaneously. There are no stops between the sets; the events are continuous.

- Take a breath; lie in the water with your face straight down. Have your right hand and arm stretched beyond your head, this is the same position as the warm-up starting position. Cup your hand (fingers at right angles to your palm, thumb pressed on your forefinger), have your left arm down by your side.

- Plunge your cupped right hand, fingers first, into the water, and start drawing it straight back in a slow curve in front of your face and chest toward your side. Exhale into the water while turning your head to the left.

- Then draw your left hand up in the air; bring your mouth into the air on the left side. You have lifted your left arm, shoulder and mouth up into the air on the same side at the same time; breathe. Have your right hand by your side.

- As you reach your left hand up past your head, turn your face back into the water; start rotating your head to the right while exhaling through your nostrils. Continue pushing your right hand toward your hip.

- Push your right hand back past your hip as far as you can to gain as much propulsion as you can from the stroke. Its force will be replaced immediately with the start of the fellow arm's stroke when you plunge your left hand into the water.

Practice every aspect until all is smooth and automatic. Don't rush it.

COMMENTS

When your hand strokes past your waist you may wish to open it while you push it toward your hip area. Changing its shape from cup to paddle may increase its propulsive effectiveness.

Stretch your legs and feet out straight to become more streamlined in the water; bent knees and standing position feet both drag.   Tense your abdominal muscles and arch your back to elevate your hips; these two adjustments could improve your streamlining when swimming.

In my opinion starting the stroke with your outstretched arm in front of your head is appropriate for the following reasons.

Not only does this stroke provide a longer propulsive pathway for your arm, but also, it may have less chance of straining a previously injured rotator cuff. This last comment is my opinion based solely on personal experience. You may wish to obtain your physician's comment on the appropriateness of this stroke to your situation.

You are by now aware of the involvement of the shoulders in swimming. The shoulder rotator cuff is part of the following story which illustrates two valuable points appropriate for those planning to re-start an exercise program.

My shoulder and neck had been injured years ago when I was thrown from a horse. An integral part of the shoulder is the rotator cuff. This complex collection of shoulder muscles, tendons, bursas and ligaments allows our great range of arm motion; re-inflaming it can result in intense pain.

I had forgotten this healed injury when I inanely challenged two of my grandsons (late teens and early 20s) to a swimming race. As you can imagine, I lost big time. What was my reward from my fierce effort: Great pain and many months of physical therapy. I had inflamed the rotator cuff in the old shoulder injury; and the following lessons I offer to you.

My first point is simple, whenever you become involved in any new exercise and feel a twinge or pain, try to recall if you ever injured that part. If you did, you may need to modify some movements involved to avoid stressing a potentially weak area. My second point is equally simple: No matter how physically improved you become you will never win when racing a younger, stronger swimmer and you probably will injure yourself. In short, don't try it.

I now turn to a harmless example of ego. As you move through the water, try to avoid or at least minimize splashing when your hands and arms enter the water. Why? Because you look better when you don't splash; take pride in your appearance.

Finally, practice. Move slowly but exactly, increase speed when each preceding rate is perfect. Then advance to the next lesson.

SECTION 4 Second Lesson: Synchronizing arm and leg movements

Introductory Comments

You should now swim somewhat automatically with your legs and feet straight out and your hips elevated. Presently, your arms and hands provide the all the forward movement; the legs only drag. The eventual goal is to add the potential power of the legs to that of the arms.

This lesson and the one that follows are linked. In this one, you will work to coordinate arm and leg movements. Two similar routines are offered. The first synchronizes fellow arms and legs; the second synchronizes opposites; try both and then choose.

This routine may take considerable concentration to perfect. During the initial learning phase wearing a snorkel mask and breathing tube may help you concentrate your actions on your legs. Later, wearing goggles, you can transfer this ability to the next and final lesson.

I have minimized the instruction details below to enhance clarity. Although I provide sets for both right and left hands, I had found when I focused on one set of arms & legs, it simplified learning because it was automatically mimicked by the other set.

Note: If you have a physical problem that prevents you from comfortably moving your hips or legs as directed in this lesson, please turn to the end of this section's primary instruction, entitled *Alternate Leg Actions*. There I suggest a few alternate moves to replace both those in this lesson and the next (Synchronizing arm and leg movements). This replacement will be the final instruction offered you in this booklet. However, please take the time to review the general information and comments in the subsequent Sections 6 & 7.

LESSON

Synchrony I

In this lesson, practice simultaneous, same side, arm and leg moves.

The following sets show paired simultaneous events, again the action is continuous.

Although it actually is simpler than it might appear, I still provide a description of the moves which begins with a basic position in the water.

- Lie in the water. Extend your right hand beyond your head; your left arm is back by your hip. Legs straight out. Begin the exercise

- Plunge your right hand in the water to start and finish a complete stroke;push your right leg up. At the same time draw your left arm out of the water and extend it past your head; push your left leg down.

- Plunge your left hand into the water to start and finish a complete stroke; force your left leg up. At the same time, draw your right arm out of the water and extend it past your head; push your right leg down.

- You have completed the first cycle of same side arms and legs.

Repeat the bulleted sections; gradually you will be able to synchronize your arm and leg moves. In my early trials I focused on my dominant arm and fellow leg initially; the other set (arm and leg) mimicked the combined movements. Gradually this will become automatic.

Synchrony II

In theory, this version should be the better of the two. It offers simultaneous forward forces on opposite sides which should result in you swimming in a straighter line. Again, action in the following sets is simultaneous, events of the sets are in sequence- there are no pauses among them.

- Lie in the water. Extend your right hand beyond your head; your left arm is back by your hip. Legs straight out. Begin the exercise:

- Plunge your right hand in the water to start and finish a complete stroke; push your left leg up, at the same time draw your left arm out of the water and extend it past your head; push your right leg down.

- Plunge your left hand into the water to start and finish a complete stroke: force your right leg up. At the same time draw your right arm out of the water and extend it past your head; push your left leg down.

You have completed the first cycle of opposite side arms and legs. Repeat the bulleted sections. Gradually you will do it automatically. Focus primarily on your dominant arm and opposite leg initially, the other set (arm and leg) will should duplicate the combined movements automatically. The aim is to train your brain in the coordination of the two arm/leg moves.

FOLLOW-UP EXERCISES

Muscle movement aids in releasing excess metabolic byproducts from exercise. In this lesson the knee is not bent thus the calf muscles do little if any contractions. As a result a buildup of by products can cause leg discomfort. To prevent or correct there are several exercises you can do: deep knee bends while in the water, flex your feet up and down 20 or so times, or do chair stands as described in Section 1.

COMMENTS

Do not seek to attain total smoothness from this lesson; its primary purpose is to enable you to synchronize arm and leg motion. Transfer this ability to the next and final lesson where you will work to synchronize and polish all your swimming moves to the best of your ability.

Alternative Leg Moves

If you found you could not perform the moves required in this lesson comfortably, select one of the following alternatives.

The one you select will be your final lesson.

First Alternative

If you have an existing problem moving your hips or feet or develop difficulty during this lesson, try the following move.

Hold your legs and feet out straight and make short up and down movements by flexing your legs at the knees. This should add some additional forward force, primarily from the soles of your feet, to that of your arms. Try to establish and maintain a rhythm. If extending your feet always causes cramping, extend them less or not at all.

Second Alternative

If you still have problems moving your legs and feet there is a simple and effective solution: hold a set of pull buoys between your calves to keep them afloat. You can find sources for this device at pool stores and on the internet under "pull buoys".

Summary for the Alternative Leg Moves

When you have attained smoothness with these alternates

you may wish to experiment with variations in arm-strokes. Those who never had a shoulder problem may wish to try the following. In this version you do not reach way out with your hand and arm, but start each stroke with your forearm at right angles to your upper arm. This stroke causes splashing on entry, but the mechanical advantage of this arm position relative to the shoulder can produce more speed; I have only observed swimmers use this stroke. This might enable you to replace the lessened or absent propulsive leg action; if you wish to try a different stroke, I suggest you search the internet.

Again, practice until it becomes automatic. You've gotten this far; work to perfect it.

SECTION 5 Third Lesson: Optimizing leg motions

Introductory Comments

This final lesson is for those who have completed the previous lesson and can synchronize arm and leg moves. As stated, one of the goals of this booklet was to offer you a method that enables you to swim gracefully and almost effortlessly.

To accomplish this I sought to minimize all possible counter- productive leg moves. In selecting them I considered several factors: the forces resulting from the positioning and movement of human legs and feet; even those of aquatic animal's limbs; the latter group produced envy. Obviously the side to side movements of fish tails were not appropriate. I attempted to try the whale-fluke movement which Michael Phelps appears to copy when he moves both legs together; it was too exhausting for this old-timer.

I completed all my deliberations, ended up selecting leg movements enhanced by gravity that accompany the efficient propulsive strokes of the arms: this upcoming method, i.e., this lesson.

FINAL LESSON   FELLOW ARMS & LEGS

Prior to this lesson, you were able to coordinate arm and leg movements and position your hips and legs near the surface of the water. Now you will work to get the most benefit from each leg movement, which is done by relaxing the appropriate leg so it sinks from the pull of gravity. This places the leg for a relatively lengthy productive upward thrust, while avoiding the effect of the unproductive downward force exerted in the previous lesson.

Action in the following sets is simultaneous, events of the sets are in sequence- there are no pauses among them.

Lie in the water, right hand forward, left hand by your hip.

- Plunge your right hand into the water to start and finish the stroke; force your right foot upward. At the same time, relax your left leg to allow it to drop; lift your left hand up, out and forward into the air to start the next stroke

- Plunge your left hand into the water to start and finish the stroke; force your left foot to the level of your body. Relax your right leg and allow it to drop. Lift your right hand up, out and forward into the air to start the next stroke.

- Repeat these steps.

Have a companion or by-stander inform you if and how much your leg has fallen. If it hasn't, work on it. Initially, this may take some concentration to achieve. The farther your leg falls, the more forward push you will obtain when you thrust it upward. Work to obtain the most amount of fall you can. Done early the maximum fall will become an automatic part of your stroke.

FINAL LESSON   OPPOSITE ARMS & LEGS

- Lie in the water, right hand forward, left hand by your hip.

- Plunge your right hand into the water to start and finish the stroke; force your left foot upward to the level of your body. At the same time, relax your right leg to allow it to drop; lift your left hand up, out and forward into the air to start the next stroke.

- Plunge your left hand into the water to start and finish the stroke; force your right foot upward to the level of your body. Relax your left leg and allow it to drop. Lift your right hand up, out and forward into the air to start the next stroke.

- Repeat these steps

FOLLOW-UP EXERCISES

You begin each swim session with warm-up exercises. The follow up exercises will enhance them to round out your routine physical activities.

Muscle groups have opposites; when you exercise one group then you should work on the other. Certain leg movements have been eliminated or minimized from these lessons because they would be counter-productive. Their effect on your body movement in the water would be an attempt to move it in an unwanted direction.

During exercise there is an increased production of metabolic by products in the associated muslce groups. Based on my observations it appears the level of these products remains high in the inactive muscle group; gradually this causes leg discomfort. Routine post-swim movements (supplemental exercises) of the formerly inactive group prevent this imbalance by utilization and elimination of these excess metabolites.

I strongly recommend you do both warm-up exercises and supplemental exercises routinely before and after each swim respectively. The best supplemental exercise is done immediately after swimming. Stand in water up to your waist and walk for several minutes or so. Force each leg forward- not backward. Others you might consider are chair stands, 10-20 done immediately after swimming; 10-20 foot flexes which can be done any time. If you do not follow this routine for exercise and experience leg discomfort, it may be relieved in several days by performing these exercises or by long walks on dry ground.

COMMENTS

Extend your arm and shoulder as far forward as possible to start each propulsive stroke. Remember to exert as much force to your arm's stroke from start to finish. Be sure that each leg is straight and your feet extended back as far as possible.

While practicing the leg coordination moves, be sure you have developed a rolling motion of your body, it should occur when the down (propulsive) stroke of one arm in water is accompanied an upward (recovery) stroke in air. These strokes assist in tilting your upper body to the 'air-side' in when your mouth is in the air. With practice this graceful motion becomes effortless and enhances awareness of nearby swimmers and objects.

While practicing one day you will experience a spontaneous spurt of speed while swimming; this rewarding sensation will occur when all your moves are synchronized as you glide through the water. Achieving this state makes all your time and efforts worthwhile, and contributes to the joy of the sport.

Swimming has improved your condition and appearance, don't let it stop there. When in or out of the water, keep your shoulders back; out of the water stand up straight. It is easier now you have been exercising. It can improve your breathing and

Swimming for the Mature Person

you'll look better.

SECTION 6 Comments about Your Skin and Swimming

Protecting against Skin Damage from the Sun

You may or may not feel you are well aware of the dangers from unprotected exposure to the sun. Now that you plan to spend time out-of-doors while swimming, the following may provide you with a little or a lot of pertinent information.

Repeated exposures of your unprotected skin to the sun can damage the skin and may eventually result in skin cancer. The danger increases as you near the equator. The damage from the UV portion of sunlight is cumulative and cannot be reversed. It will happen to any unprotected person who ventures out during the day, even when it is overcast.

Take protective steps each time you swim out of doors during the day. Limit further damage by controlling exposure time and also by the liberal application of UV sun blockers. The World Health Organization advises avoiding exposure to the sun after 10AM, and before 4PM; most especially when the sun is directly overhead. Apply a recognized brand of water-proof sun block with a high SPF (Sun Protection Factor) value. Even when you are coated with sun blocker the duration of exposure probably is best limited to about a half hour, with possibly somewhat longer exposures at the beginning and end of the day. Wear wide- brimmed hats for out-of- pool protection.

Use water-proof sun blockers: Coppertone Sport Sunblock® is one example, Bull Frog® is another. For a more complete listing of products check on the internet under sun block or sunscreen for swimmers. Some are available as creams or gels, others as aerosol sprays. I have found by using an aerosol dispenser I can spray my own back while resorting to minimal gymnastics. Do not spray a blocker on your face, nor apply a cream version near your eyes. The blocker can 'walk' onto the surface of your eyes from lid movement or be washed in with perspiration; you will sense the irritation shortly afterwards. Besides, that area probably does need extra protection while you are swimming face down and wearing goggles.

As one who now spends more time in the sun, you must also reckon with photosensitivity from certain drugs that will cause you to burn on minimal exposure to the sun. It is possible that your physician may direct you to avoid any exposure to the sun while on certain medications, if not, it may be prudent to limit your out-of-door swimming to the early morning or late afternoon even when coated with a sun blocker when taking these drugs. Examples of these drugs are sulfas, certain diuretics and the tetracyclines. Check your prescription labels for these warnings: usually such information is provided on the prescription container or in the accompanying information sheet. If not, you can find information from your pharmacist, physician or on the internet.

The bald and those with shaved heads should also wear UV protective bathing caps. Properly worn they can cover both scalp and ears. When you swim in the ocean, I suggest you wear a yellow cap; it will not only protect your scalp but will enhance your detection from shore when needed.

Remember to wear quality, protective sunglasses; your skin is not the only part of you that it damaged by solar UV.

Swimmer's Ear

Swimmer's ear is a common problem. Reportedly, it is a minor fungal infection of the external ear canal. This is not surprising when you consider how well fungus grows in warm, moist areas.

Years ago, after my case had been treated with a series of prescription ear drops. I was seen by an ear specialist (otolaryngologist). He provided me with a simple formula for a home-made ear drop I still use. It is a mixture of white vinegar and rubbing alcohol 50:50. For my use, I select an empty dropper bottle previously containing an Rx or OTC nose or eye drop, thoroughly clean the bottle and tip, and then fill it with the mixture.

To prevent its misuse apply an indelible labeling to the container that states clearly that the contents are only for use in the ear. Although it is comfortable in the ear canal, it is slightly irritating when it spills out onto the cheek so have a tissue handy to blot any excess. I have used the vinegar-alcohol mixture after swimming even after the irritation cleared to remove water trapped in my ears.

Warning: the vinegar/alcohol mixture is only for ears with non- perforated ear drums and must never be used in the eye or the nose. If by chance some were to get into the eyes it would require immediate require rinsing out with copious volumes of water, e.g. hose, faucet or a leap into the pool.

If it causes any more than temporary visual problems seek medical treatment. Last but not least, keep it out of reach of children or the poorly sighted. Obviously, if you have a condition that does not respond promptly to this simple treatment, see a physician promptly. *Be sure to read the statement at the end of this section regarding the use of this formulation and other items mentioned.*

Swimmer's Itch

There are two categories of swimmer's itch: The first is a skin infection from swimming in polluted lake or pond water; the second is an irritation caused by chlorine in pool water. The first is beyond the scope of this booklet; I shall discuss the second; itching caused by chlorinated water.

Many people are hyper-sensitive to chlorine in water. It ranges from a problem with contact of any part of their skin with chlorinated water including the small concentration in tap water; this problem is common enough that dechlorinating shower heads are available. Those extremely sensitive persons are not the subject of this section.

Swimmer's itch affects some areas of swimmer's skin those who routinely come in contact with the more concentrated chlorine of swimming pools. This annoying itch does not affect the entire skin, but develops gradually in relatively small areas of the skin. It first appears after even several days or more and becomes intolerable. For us the itch resisted applications of OTC and Rx strength hydrocortisone cream, pretreatment with antihistamines and neutralization with a chlorine neutralizing product such as UltraSwim®. It seemed as if the only answers were to either swim in non-chlorinated or quit swimming.

My wife and I finally gained total relief by the application of a skin smoothing lotion: Lubriderm® Advanced Therapy Smoothing Lotion with active AHA. She had purchased it after being diagnosed with a dry skin condition; she luckily picked up this specific version of the product, i.e., with AHA (Alpha Hydroxy Acid). We use it as follows. Right after the post-swim shower we apply it only to the affected areas while they are still wet. We re-apply it later if there is some residual itching (re-moisten the skin for easier spreading of the lotion). We limit the application to the relatively small affected areas. We are aware of the labeling that advised the AHA can increase the danger of sunburn and routinely apply a water-proof sunscreen (SPF 50-70) to all exposed skin.

To the best of my knowledge the manufacturer of Lubriderm® Advanced Therapy Smoothing Lotion with active AHA has neither submitted it to, nor gained approval from the US Food and Drug Administration (FDA) for the prevention and or treatment of swimmer's itch. Be sure to read and understand the labeling, especially the SUNBURN ALERT. It states that the AHA ingredient may increase your skin's sensitivity to the sun and with it the possibility of sunburn. It states that one should use a sunscreen, protective clothing and limit exposure to the sun during its use and for a week following. I called the number listed on the label and spoke with the manufacturer's agent about precautions. She informed me that all one need do is cover the area where the lotion had been applied with a sunscreen prior to exposure to the sun.

Important Note

Please read and understand the following regarding the alcohol/vinegar ear drops and any commercially available product mentioned in this booklet.

I have neither conducted,nor read any formal scientific research regarding any of these items as remedies – accordingly, I can offer no assurance that any will be safe and effective in your case. I am simply recounting my own experience for whatever interest it may have. You are encouraged to make whatever inquiries you think necessary or prudent.

SECTION 7 Summary Comments

Check List

Re-evaluate your swimming occasionally; I suggest you use the following list.

- Warm-up exercises

- Face in 'breathing position' at each stroke, even at times

- when you do not take a breath.

- Each arm and shoulder extended from far forward to

- backwards as possible; entire stroke done forcefully.

- Legs straight; feet pointed back; moves synchronized with

- arms. Force each upward stroke.

- Hips kept as close as possible to the surface of the water.

- Supplemental leg exercises

Ocean Swimming

In the ocean, waves and current direction are rarely consistent or cooperative with the swimmer. Unless you are trying out for the Olympics you can obtain adequate exercise swimming near or parallel to the shore.

If you can only breathe on one side, you will have a problem when the waves prevent you from swimming in the only direction to safety. I was once in this predicament. I had planned to describe the actions I took, but when recalling the details I am sure my survival was mainly luck not skill. My heartfelt advice: When swimming in the ocean stay near the shore or near an accessible boat.

I have read that sharks are most active early and late in the day when the light level is minimal. Avoid wearing shiny jewelry or other reflective items; reports indicate that these animals are attracted by any light-reflector. Be mindful that they may without malice mistake a reflection from your watch or jewelry as originating from a tasty fish's scales. This could be unfortunate.

Linear Lap Swimming

If you have a problem swimming in a straight line and occasionally collide with other swimmers or protruding sections of pool walls, etc., I have a possible solution to your problem. Purchase a length of dark colored 3/8" or so wide chain and lay it along the bottom of the pool. It can serve as a marker line for lap swimmers. I found it best when the chain is shorter than the pool by a few feet on either end; this could warn you that you are approaching the end of the pool and save you from swimming into it.

If you must remove and store the chain after each session, you can avoid snarls by winding it around a discarded chain or wire spool. Discarded spools are usually available from a hardware dealer. Note: unspooled painted metal chains can leave rust marks when stored wet; if you feel this will be a problem, purchase plastic chains. If you own your own pool, avoid all this by having lap lines painted on the bottom.

Persistence

To anyone who has read this far and it still not convinced that swimming is the way, read on. Let me try one more to convince you to never give up on the goal of swimming for exercise and entertainment. People have gone to remarkable degrees to overcome problems so they can swim. Consider the following two.

I knew one indomitable lady who was born without arms. She swam regularly; she moved so well through the water that inconsiderate swimmers would occasionally forget her situation, whereupon they would receive her genteel wrath after they had splashed water in her face. In September 2010, Philippe Croizon a 42-year old who had lost much of both arms and legs, had himself fitted with flippers. Later he swam the English Channel.

Croizon's choice of swimming venue would not be mine, but both people's persistence diminishes our relatively trivial excuses for not swimming.

To the reader who used to swim but doesn't anymore, reconsider. In some cases the decision not to swim is a psychological, not a physical item that need to be overcome.

From experience I can predict from time to time you will have an overwhelming urge to forego leaving the comfort of your home for your regular swim. The reasons are predictable and trivial: The outside temperature is not suitable, you're just feeling lazy, etc. Force yourself to get up and go. During and following the swim, you will be elated, refreshed, and once more happy that you did not procrastinate. This I know from experience.

Final Statement

I hope you have enjoyed and benefited from the booklet. Self- taught swimming brought my wife and me into this sport we have relished for nearly a quarter of a century. We often reflect on the various places around the globe where we have enjoyed this sport; they have ranged from the mundane to the exotic to the remarkable. Each swim was exhilarating. We reflected on the various pools we had enjoyed; two came to mind because of their unusual cylindrical configurations. One was in an Amsterdam airport hotel bar, the other of volcanic origin was off the shore of Molokai in Hawaii. But each provided an enjoyable site for swimming. Hopefully you will visit many diverse venues where you can practice this salubrious sport.

The author wishes to thank Dawn MacKeen for her review.

swim@mackeen.com

68

www.ingramcontent.com/pod-product-compliance
Lightning Source LLC
Chambersburg PA
CBHW021248280526
45784CB00005B/2283